Copyright

Esther Campbell

Table of contents

Introduction

A. Importance of Exercise for Seniors Over 60. In the golden years of life, being active is not simply an option; it's a crucial necessity. The benefits of exercise for adults over 60 cannot be overemphasized. As the years pass, our bodies naturally undergo changes, but this doesn't imply we should slow down and maintain a sedentary lifestyle. Quite the reverse, in fact. Regular exercise is the key to maintaining physical and mental health as we age. In this book, we'll explore how easy and pleasurable activities may alter your life, no matter your age or current fitness level.

B. **Benefits of Staying Active in Your 60s**.

Why should you bother with fitness in your 60s? The benefits are enormous and life-changing. Staying active in your 60s can help you maintain and perhaps improve your overall health and well-being. From increased cardiovascular health and stronger muscles to improved balance and flexibility, exercise can empower you to lead a more independent and satisfying life. Beyond the physical rewards, exercise also plays a significant role in boosting mental clarity, lowering stress, and creating a happy outlook on life. Through this book, we will explore how these benefits are within your reach, regardless of your starting point.

C. **Purpose of the Book**.

This book is exclusively developed for seniors over 60 who desire a comprehensive reference to safe, effective, and entertaining workouts customized to their age group. Whether you're a seasoned fitness enthusiast or someone who's never engaged in organized exercise before, you'll discover essential knowledge and inspiration inside these pages. Our mission is to enable you to take control of your health and vitality, proving that it's never too late to start or enhance your fitness journey. We aim to provide you with practical guidance, fitness routines, and encouragement to enjoy a healthier, more active, and happier life in your 60s and beyond.

Now, let's go on this adventure together, covering a wide selection of activities and tactics that will enable you to make the most of this exciting era of life. Whether you're wanting to maintain your current level of fitness or begin a new journey, this book is your trusted guide on the route to a healthier and more active self.

Chapter 1

Types of Exercises

A. Aerobic Exercises

1. **Walking**: Walking is one of the easiest yet most efficient cardio workouts for seniors. It's easy on the joints and can be done practically anywhere, making it a great choice. Regular walking helps improve cardiovascular health, strengthens leg muscles, and enhances overall stamina. Start with shorter walks

and progressively increase your duration to enjoy the best benefits.

2. **Swimming**: Swimming delivers a low-impact, full-body workout that's gentle on the joints. It's a fantastic choice for seniors with joint pain or arthritis. The buoyancy of water lessens the chance of injury while providing resistance for muscular toning. Swimming also improves flexibility and encourages relaxation.

3. **Cycling**: Cycling is a terrific way to get your heart beating and your legs moving.

Whether on a stationary bike or a normal bicycle, cycling helps increase cardiovascular fitness and lower body strength. It's a versatile exercise that allows you to pick the intensity and length that suit your fitness level.

B. **Strength Training**

1. **Bodyweight Exercises**: Bodyweight exercises, such as squats, lunges, and push-ups, use your own body weight as resistance. These workouts help build and maintain muscle mass, promote

bone density, and improve overall strength. They can be modified to your fitness level and completed in the comfort of your home.

2. **Resistance Band Workouts**: Resistance bands are lightweight and portable instruments that are great for seniors. They provide resistance throughout the range of action, making it easier to target specific muscle groups. Resistance band workouts can enhance muscle strength, flexibility, and balance

while lowering the risk of injury associated with lifting large weights.

C. **Flexibility and Balance Exercises**

1. **Yoga**:

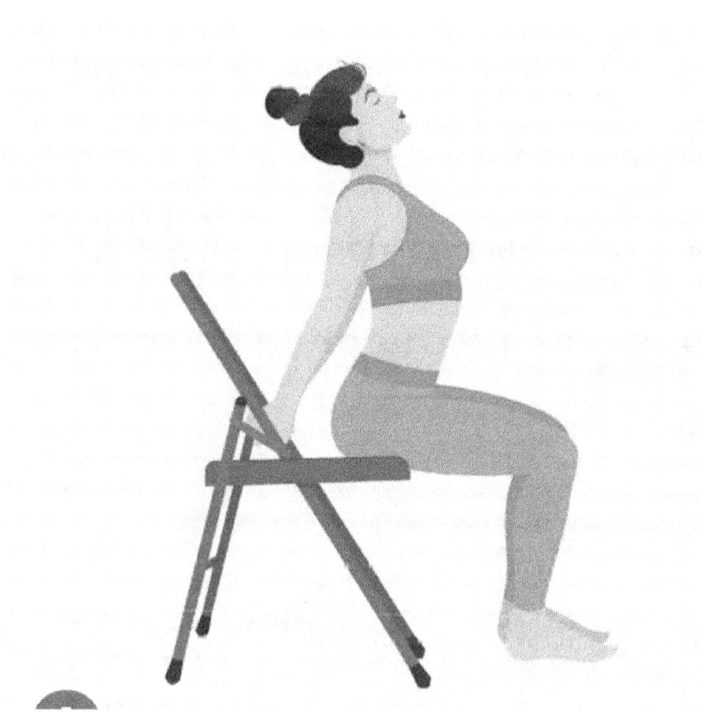

Yoga is a peaceful yet powerful exercise that blends stretching, balance, and mindfulness. It boosts flexibility, improves posture, and helps alleviate aches and pains. Yoga also improves relaxation and reduces stress, making it a wonderful alternative for seniors wishing to improve both physical and mental well-being.

Examples of yoga exercises for elders over 60:

1. **Mountain Pose (Tadasana):**

Stand with your feet hip-width apart.

Roll your shoulders back and down

.Keep your arms loose at your sides.

Focus on your breath and feel grounded, like a mountain.

2. Chair Pose (Utkatasana):

Stand with your feet hip-width apart and your arms at your sides. Inhale and raise your arms overhead. Exhale, bend your knees, and drop your hips as if sitting in a chair. Keep your weight in your heels and your chest elevated. Hold for a few breaths and gently return to a standing position.

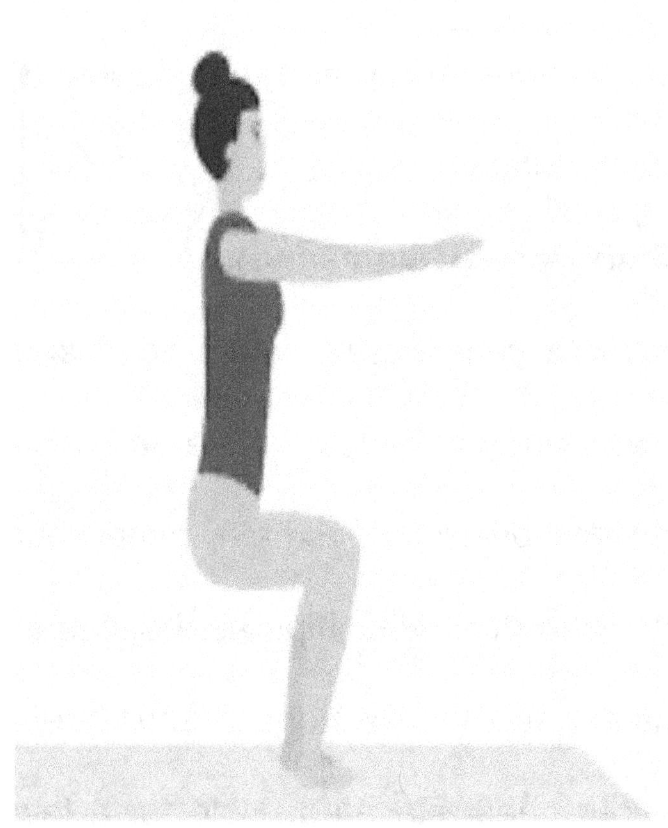

3. **Cat-Cow Stretch:**

Beggin on your hands and knees in a tabletop position. Inhale and arch your back, elevating your head and tailbone (Cow Pose). Exhale, rounding your spine and tucking your chin (Cat Pose). Repeat this slow flow, matching breath with movement.

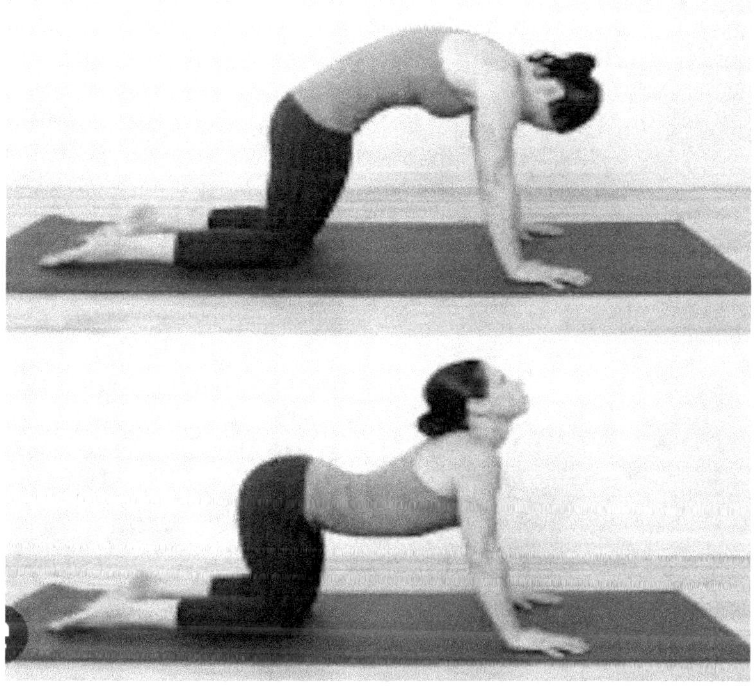

4. **Legs Up the Wall (Viparita Karani):**

Sit with your back against a wall. Swing your legs up the wall while resting on your back. Keep your legs straight or with a slight bend. Relax your arms at your sides.

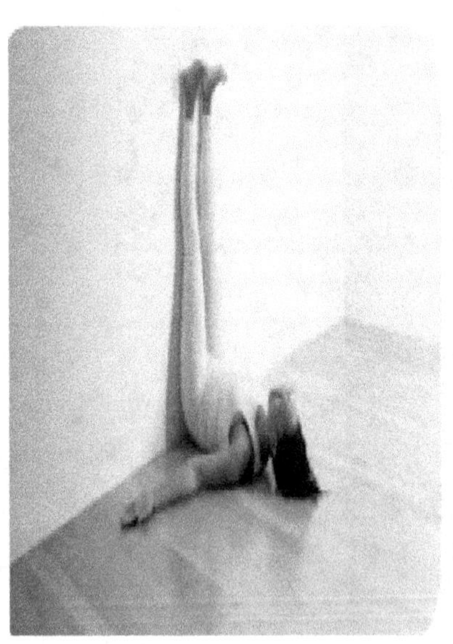 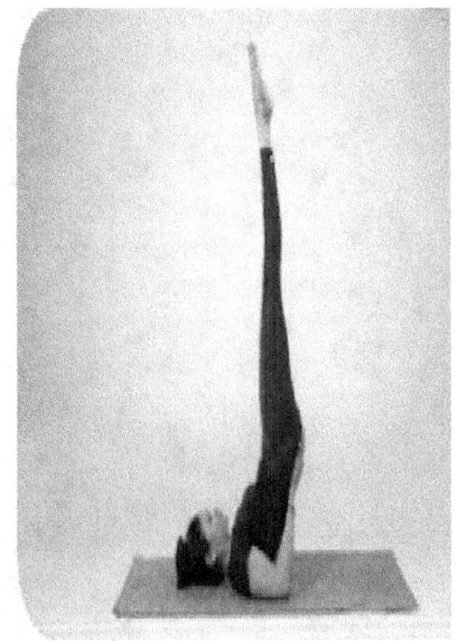

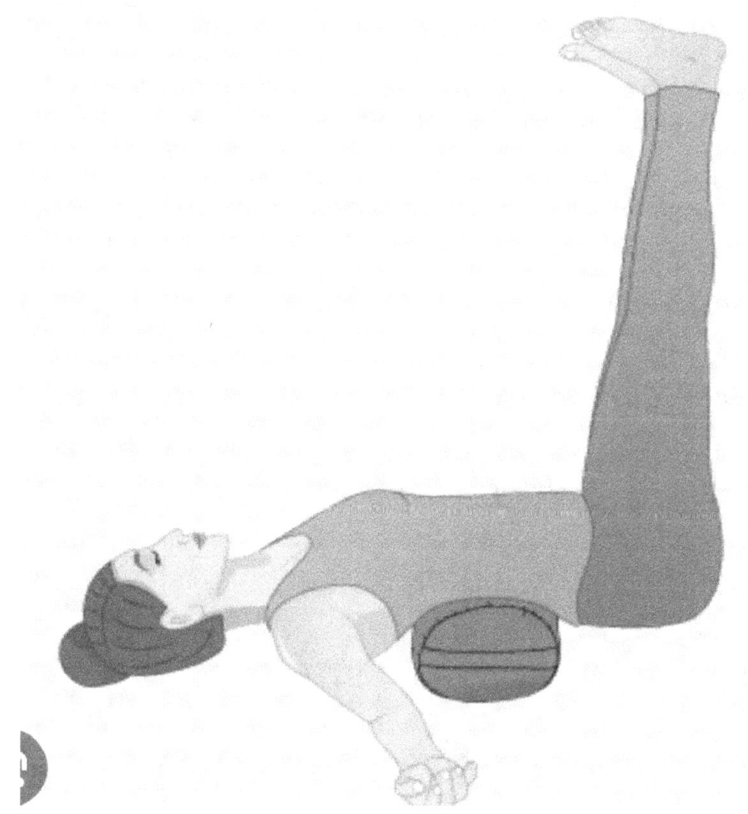

5. **Seated Forward Bend** (Paschimottanasana):

Sit with your legs out in front of you.Inhale and stretch your spine.Exhale, hinge at your hips, and extend forward toward your toes.If you can't reach your toes, grab your ankles or shins.Keep your back straight and avoid rounding.Hold for a few breaths, and then slowly release.These yoga techniques enhance flexibility, balance, and relaxation without putting excessive strain on the body. Always practice at your own pace and alter poses as needed to match your comfort and abilities.

2. **Tai Chi:**

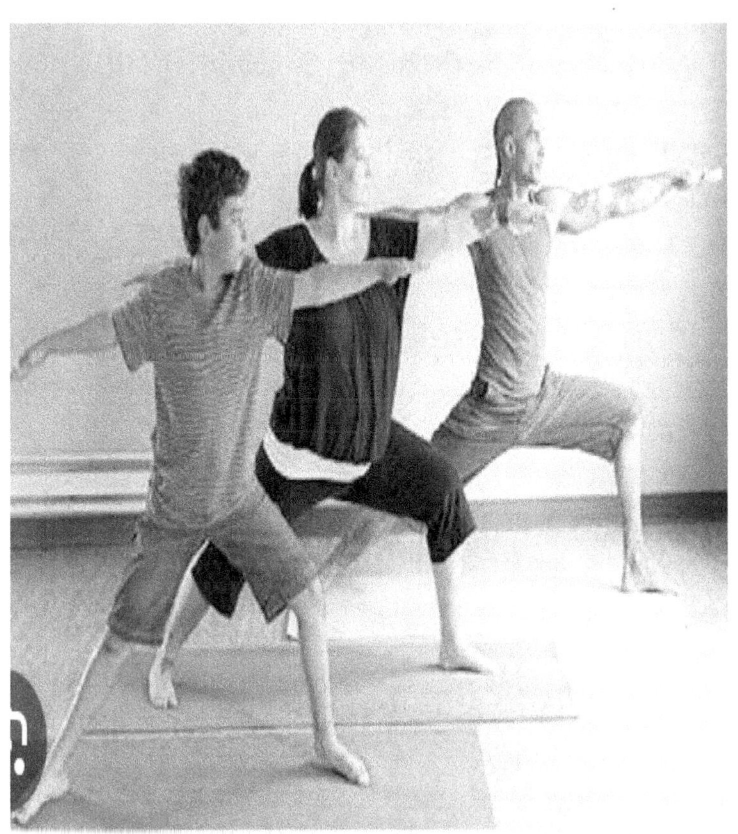

Tai Chi is a gentle and graceful martial technique that stresses balance, coordination, and flowing motions. It's particularly good for elders as it minimizes the chance of falls, promotes flexibility, and cultivates a sense of peace. Regular Tai Chi practice can enhance general physical and mental equilibrium.

Tai Chi workouts are gentle and excellent for seniors over 60. Here are three Tai Chi exercises suitable for this age group:

Brush your knee and push forward.

Start with your feet shoulder-width apart, knees slightly bent, and arms relaxed at your sides. Shift your weight onto one leg while simultaneously elevating the opposing hand. As you shift your weight back to center, spin your hand and arm, brushing them across your torso. Simultaneously, step forward with the leg on the side of the lifted hand and softly push forward. Repeat this action on both sides in a slow and controlled manner, syncing with your breath. Grasp the Sparrow's Tail:

Begin with your feet shoulder-width apart. Raise both arms in front of you, palms facing each other. As you exhale, open one arm to the side, twisting your torso.

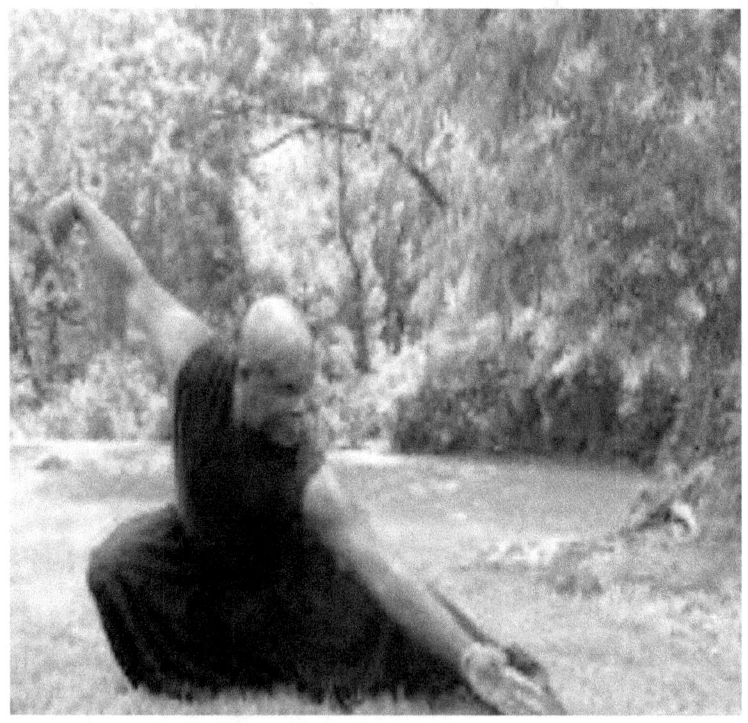

Inhale as you bring the open arm back to the center. Exhale again as you push the second arm to the side, twisting your torso in the opposite direction. Continue this smooth, flowing movement, like a bird spreading its wings and then folding them back.

Wave Hands in Clouds:

Start with your feet shoulder-width apart, knees slightly bent, and arms relaxed at your sides. Shift your weight to one side while twisting your torso slightly. Begin a continuous, flowing motion with your arms: one hand rises while the other descends. As you shift your weight to the opposite side, reverse the arm movement. The arms should move in a circular, cloud-like pattern. Continue this graceful, flowing movement for several repetitions on each side.

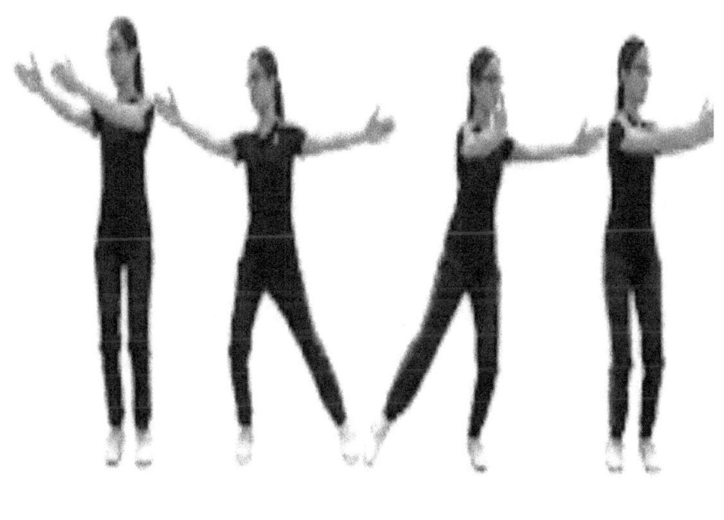

Tai Chi exercises promote balance, flexibility, and relaxation, making them an excellent choice for seniors looking to improve physical and mental well-being.

These exercises are typically performed slowly and mindfully, focusing on the coordination of breath and movement. Remember to practice at your own pace and consult with a certified Tai Chi instructor for proper guidance and form.

3. **Stretching Routines:**

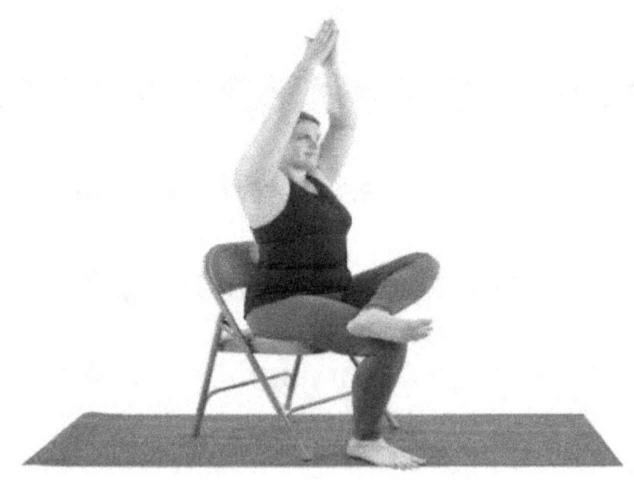

Stretching exercises, whether standalone or incorporated into your daily routine, help maintain and improve flexibility. Stretching routines can target specific muscle groups, relieving tension and reducing the risk of injuries. They are especially important for seniors to maintain mobility and prevent stiffness. Incorporating a variety of these exercises into your fitness regimen can provide a well-rounded approach to staying active and healthy as a senior.

Chapter 2

Exercise Routines

A. Weekly Exercise Plans

Sample Schedules:

Creating a weekly activity schedule is vital for remaining on track with your fitness goals. Here are two sample schedules to help you get started:

Sample Schedule

 1 (Moderate Intensity):

Monday: 30 minutes of brisk walking

Tuesday: 20 minutes of bodyweight workouts (e.g., squats, push-ups)

Wednesday: Rest day

Thursday: 20 minutes of swimming or water aerobics.

Friday: 30 minutes of cycling

Saturday: 20 minutes of Tai Chi

Sunday: Rest day Sample Schedule 2 (Gentle Routine):

Monday: 15 minutes of stretching and relaxation (e.g., yoga)

Tuesday: 20 minutes of resistance band workouts

Wednesday: Rest day

Thursday: 20 minutes of low-impact aerobics

Friday: 15 minutes of balance exercises (e.g., Tai Chi)

Saturday: 30 minutes of walking

Sunday: Rest day

Customizing Routines: Your weekly workout routine should be personalized to your unique fitness level, goals, and any existing health issues. If you have special health concerns, talk with a healthcare expert or a fitness trainer to build a customized strategy. Remember that it's crucial to start cautiously and gradually increase the intensity and duration of your activities as your fitness improves.

B. **Demonstrations and Instructions**

Step-by-Step Guidance:

Detailed, step-by-step guidance is crucial for elders to execute exercises effectively and securely. Each exercise in your routine should be presented fully, including proper posture, movement, and breathing techniques. Visual tools, such as diagrams or movies, can be particularly helpful in illustrating perfect form.

Proper Form and Safety Tips: Ensuring proper form is vital for preventing injuries. Include safety tips for each exercise, such as:

Maintain proper posture and alignment.Start with modest resistance or weight, then gradually increase it.Use steady support if needed (e.g., a chair for balance).Listen to your body, and stop if you encounter pain or discomfort.Stay hydrated throughout your workout.Warm up before exercising and cool down afterward. Additionally, give advice on adaptations and alternatives for exercises so seniors with various abilities can participate safely. Encourage the use of safety equipment, including comfortable training shoes and resistance bands, to enhance the exercise experience.

Chapter 3

Overcoming Challenges

A. Dealing with Common Health Concerns

Arthritis: Arthritis is a major worry among seniors, causing joint discomfort and stiffness. To address this challenge:

Consult with a healthcare provider to establish safe exercises and adaptations. Focus on low-impact activities like swimming, Tai Chi, or stationary cycling.Use mild range-of-motion exercises to maintain joint flexibility.Apply heat or cold therapy as prescribed for pain relief.

Osteoporosis: Seniors with osteoporosis suffer a higher risk of fractures.

Here's how to deal with it:

Incorporate weight-bearing workouts like walking, dancing, or resistance training to improve bone density.

Ensure a diet rich in calcium and vitamin D to maintain bone health.

Perform balance and posture exercises to prevent falls.

Joint Pain: Joint pain can be caused by several sources, including arthritis or overuse.

To manage joint pain:

Prioritize low-impact workouts to reduce pressure on the joints.

Apply mild stretches and warm-up activities before activities. Consider anti-inflammatory drugs if suggested by a healthcare expert.

B. Motivation and Consistency

Staying Inspired: Staying inspired is vital for a persistent workout. Try these strategies:

Set specific and achievable goals, whether it's improving flexibility, decreasing weight, or increasing endurance. Find a workout buddy or join group courses for social support. Vary your routine to keep things fresh and prevent boredom. Reward yourself for reaching milestones, such as by treating yourself to a favorite nutritious snack or a relaxing bath.

Tracking Progress: Tracking your progress can enhance motivation and help you see your achievements. Here's how:

Maintain an activity notebook to track your workouts, including time and intensity. Use fitness apps or wearable devices to measure your steps, heart rate, and other parameters. Periodically measure your fitness level with easy tests like evaluating your flexibility or documenting how many push-ups you can perform. Celebrate tiny successes and acknowledge gains in your general health, even if they're gradual. Remember that failures might happen, but they don't define your fitness path. Stay patient and adaptive, changing your schedule as needed to accommodate changes in your health or circumstances. By addressing common health concerns and sustaining enthusiasm, you may overcome hurdles and make exercise a sustainable part of your life, reaping the many benefits it brings to seniors over 60.

Chapter 4

Nutrition and Hydration

A. The Importance of a Healthy Diet

Maintaining a nutritious diet is crucial for adults over 60. A balanced diet delivers the vital elements necessary for optimum health and well-being.

Nutrient Density: As you age, your body's nutrient requirements remain high, but your calorie needs may drop. Therefore, it's crucial to consume nutrient-dense foods that provide vitamins, minerals, fiber, and protein without unnecessary calories.

Strong Bones: Adequate calcium and vitamin D intake is crucial for bone health, especially to battle osteoporosis.

Heart Health: A diet rich in fruits, vegetables, whole grains, and lean proteins can help maintain healthy blood pressure and cholesterol levels, minimizing the risk of cardiovascular disease.

Weight Management: Maintaining a healthy weight is vital to preventing obesity-related health concerns. A balanced diet aids in weight control and helps manage chronic illnesses like diabetes.

Digestive Health: Fiber from fruits, vegetables, and whole grains supports digestive regularity by avoiding constipation and aiding in nutrient absorption.

B. **Hydration Tips for Seniors**

Proper hydration is equally crucial for elders, as aging can reduce the body's ability to perceive thirst. Here are some hydration tips:

Drink Water Regularly: Aim to drink water frequently throughout the day, even if you don't feel thirsty. Pale yellow or light straw-colored urine is an indication of appropriate hydration, but dark yellow or amber pee may indicate dehydration.

Limit Caffeine and Alcohol: Both caffeine and alcohol can have diuretic effects, raising the risk of dehydration.

Eat water-rich foods: Incorporate foods with high water content, such as fruits (e.g., watermelon, oranges) and vegetables (e.g., cucumber, lettuce), into your meals and snacks.

Stay mindful of drugs. Some drugs may induce excessive urination or impair fluid balance.

Address Special Needs: Seniors with special health conditions, like kidney troubles, may require individualized hydration strategies.

Adjust for climate and exertion: Hot weather, strenuous exertion, or illness might increase fluid demands. Be mindful of these things and adjust your water consumption accordingly.

Chapter 5

Mind-Body Connection

A. Relaxation Techniques

Meditation:

Meditation is a powerful technique that increases the mind-body connection by encouraging relaxation and reducing stress. Here's how it works:

Find a quiet and comfortable location to sit or lie down. Focus your attention on your breath, a mantra, or a tranquil image. As thoughts arise, recognize them without judgment and gently redirect your focus to your selected area of concentration. Regular meditation can help reduce anxiety, improve sleep, and develop mindfulness, promoting a sense of inner calm and well-being.

Deep Breathing: Deep breathing techniques, also known as diaphragmatic breathing, improve relaxation by soothing the nervous system.

To practice deep breathing:

Sit or lie down in a comfortable position. Inhale gently and deeply through your nose, allowing your abdomen to rise.

Exhale slowly and completely through your mouth, letting go of stress with each breath. Repeat this procedure for many minutes, focusing on your breath and letting go of stress.

B. **Mental Exercises**

Brain Games: Engaging in brain games like crossword puzzles, Sudoku, or chess can be pleasant and healthy for cognitive health. These activities challenge memory, problem-solving skills, and strategic thinking. Regularly participating in brain games can help you maintain mental sharpness and cognitive performance as you age.

Cognitive Challenges: Beyond games, cognitive challenges involve tasks that stimulate your thinking and learning abilities. Consider activities such as:

Learning a new language or musical instrument Engaging in creative activities like painting, writing, or crafting. Taking up educational courses or workshops. Exploring new subjects or reading books on varied topics. Solving riddles or puzzles that involve critical thought. These activities keep your brain busy and adaptive, helping to minimize cognitive decline and promote mental agility. The mind-body link is reinforced when you engage in activities that promote both mental and emotional well-being. By combining relaxation techniques and mental exercises into your daily routine, you can establish a better balance between your mental and physical health, leading to a more rewarding and peaceful life as you age.

Chapter 6

Social and Community Engagement

A. Group Exercise Classes

Participating in group exercise courses can be a terrific way for seniors over 60 to be active and socially involved.

Here's why:

Motivation and Accountability: Group sessions provide a motivating environment where you're surrounded by like-minded individuals working towards similar fitness goals. The companionship and friendly competition can inspire you to stay regular with your fitness program.

Structured Workouts: Group sessions frequently follow a structured training plan supervised by experienced instructors. This guarantees that you engage in a well-rounded exercise plan that addresses multiple facets of health, from cardiovascular fitness to strength and flexibility.

Social Interaction: Attending regular sessions allows you to meet and interact with people who share your interests. Building friendships inside the class can make exercise more pleasurable and lead to enduring social connections.

B. **Building a Support System**

Building a support system is vital for sustaining physical and emotional well-being as a senior. Here's how to go about it:

Family and Friends: Stay connected with family and friends who provide emotional support and company. Share your fitness journey with them, and you might even inspire them to join you in remaining active.

Join Clubs and Organizations: Explore local clubs or organizations that correspond with your interests, whether it's a hiking club, a gardening group, or a reading club. These communities provide the opportunity to mingle while pursuing shared passions.

Online Communities: The internet offers a multitude of online communities and forums focusing on numerous themes, including health and wellness for seniors. These virtual spaces can provide a sense of belonging and support, especially if in-person connections are restricted.

C. Staying socially active

Maintaining an active social life is vital for mental and emotional well-being in your 60s and beyond.

Attend social events: participate in social events such as family gatherings, community meetings, or local events and festivals. These occasions provide an opportunity to engage with others and share experiences.

Volunteer: Volunteering for local charities or groups can be a gratifying way to keep socially engaged while giving back to the community. Volunteering also delivers a sense of purpose and fulfillment.

Embrace Technology: Utilize technology to stay in touch with loved ones, especially if they are geographically distant. Video conversations, social media, and messaging apps can help bridge the gap and preserve ties.

Explore New Interests: Pursue new hobbies or interests that include social contact. Whether it's taking a dance class, joining a sports league, or attending workshops, attempting something new might lead to meeting like-minded others.

Conclusion

A. Recap of Key PointsIn this thorough guide on exercises for seniors over 60, we've addressed the value of remaining active, the numerous types of workouts accessible, tactics to overcome common health concerns, ways to stay motivated, and the significance of adequate nutrition and hydration. We've also delved into the mind-body connection and the benefits of social and community engagement. Let's recall the major takeaways:

Exercise is crucial for sustaining physical and mental health in your 60s and beyond. Aerobic workouts, weight training, flexibility, and balance exercises create a well-rounded fitness plan. Customizing your fitness routine is vital to accommodating individual demands and preferences. Dealing with common health conditions, including arthritis, osteoporosis, and joint discomfort, requires personalized approaches. Staying motivated and tracking progress are key to long-term consistency. A balanced diet and sufficient hydration complement your fitness endeavors. The mind-body connection, including relaxation techniques and mental exercises, contributes to general well-being. Social and community engagement boost both physical and emotional health.

B. **Encouragement for a Healthier Future.**

It's never too late to pursue a better, more active lifestyle. As you move forward, remember that consistency is vital. Small, steady changes can lead to big increases in your well-being. Keep your goals in mind and stay inspired by the wonderful influence exercise and a healthy lifestyle can have on your life.

Embrace the thrill of movement and choose things that offer you satisfaction. Whether it's a regular walk, a group workout class, or a new interest, make fitness a part of your daily routine. Cherish the sense of accomplishment that comes with each step you take towards a healthy future.

C. **Additional Resources and References.**

To continue your path towards improved health, consider exploring other resources and references. These can include:

Books and articles about elder exercise, nutrition, and well-being. Online communities and forums where you can connect with like-minded individuals.

Local fitness establishments, senior centers, or community organizations offer exercise programs specialized for seniors.

Appendices:

A. Exercise Log Templates

Keeping a record of your exercise routines can help you stay accountable and track your progress.

Here are two exercise log templates you can use:

1. Weekly Exercise Log:

Day	Activit y	Durati on	Intensi ty	Notes

Mon.				
Tues.				
Wed.				
Thurs.				
Fri.				
Sat.				
Sun.				

2. Progress Tracker:

Date	Weight (lbs)	Waist circumstance (inches)	Fitness goals	Achievement
dd/mm/yyyy				

dd/m m/yyy y				
dd/m m/yyy y				

B. Recommended Reading List

Expand your knowledge of senior fitness and well-being with these recommended reading materials:

"Younger Next Year: Live Strong, Fit, and Sexy - Until You're 80 and Beyond" by Chris Crowley and Henry S. Lodge, M.D.

"The Blue Zones: 9 Lessons for Living Longer From the People Who've Lived the Longest" by Dan Buettner.

"Strength Training Past 50" by Wayne L. Westcott and Thomas R. Baechle.

"The New Rules of Lifting for Life: An All-New Muscle-Building, Fat-Blasting Plan for Men and Women Who Want to Ace Their Midlife Exams" by Lou Schuler and Alwyn Cosgrove.

"Chair Yoga: Sit, Stretch, and Strengthen Your Way to a Happier, Healthier You" by Kristin McGee.

C. Useful Websites and Apps

Explore these online resources and mobile applications to further support your journey to better health:

Websites:

National Institute on Aging - Exercise and Physical Activity

SilverSneakers

My Fitness Pal - A comprehensive app and website for tracking nutrition and exercise.

Apps:

MyFitnessPal (iOS/Android) - Easily track your food intake and exercise, set goals, and connect with a supportive community.

Fitbod (iOS/Android) - Generate personalized workout plans based on your fitness goals and available equipment.

Calm (iOS/Android) - A meditation and relaxation app to reduce stress and improve mindfulness.

Yoga for Beginners (iOS/Android) - Access beginner-friendly yoga routines and tutorials to improve flexibility and balance.

These resources can provide additional guidance, motivation, and support as you work towards a healthier and more active lifestyle in your 60s and beyond.

9 798860 118485